The Vibrant Lean and Green Cookbook

Delicious and Healthy Recipes to Stay Fit and Boost
Your Taste

Lyman Price

Table of contents

Apple Crisp

Prep Time: 15 minutes.

Cook Time: 40 minutes.

Serves: 4

Ingredients:

- 4 cups apples, peeled and sliced
- 1 tablespoon coconut oil, melted
- 1/2 teaspoon cinnamon
- 1/4 teaspoon ground ginger

Crisp Topping

- ½ teaspoon cinnamon
- ¼ teaspoon ginger
- ¼ teaspoon nutmeg
- 1 cup old fashioned oats
- 1/3 cup pecans chopped
- 2 tablespoons coconut oil
- 1 tablespoon maple syrup

Preparation:

1. At 350 degrees F, preheat your oven. Grease an 8x8 inch baking dish.
2. Toss apples with coconut oil, ginger and cinnamon in a bowl.
3. Spread the apples in the baking dish.

4. Mix all the crisp topping in a bowl and drizzle over the apples.

5. Cover this baking dish with aluminium foil and bake for 20 minutes at 350 degrees F.

6. Uncover the hot dish and bake for another 20 minutes.

7. Serve.

Serving Suggestion: Serve the apple crisp with chopped nuts on top.

Variation Tip: Add dried raisins to the apple crisp.

Nutritional Information Per Serving:

Calories 203 | Fat 8.9g |Sodium 340mg | Carbs 24.7g | Fiber 1.2g | Sugar 11.3g | Protein 5.3g

Cherry Dessert

Prep Time: 15 minutes.

 Cook Time: 0 minutes.

Serves: 4

Ingredients:

- 2 cups lite whipped topping, thawed
- 1 (8-ounce) package cream cheese, softened
- 1 package sugar-free cherry gelatin
- 1/2 cup boiling water

Preparation:

1. Beat cream with cream cheese in a bowl until smooth.
2. Mix gelatin mix with boiling water in a bowl.
3. Add this prepared gelatin mixture to the cream cheese mixture.
4. Mix well and spread this mixture into a pie pan.
5. Cover and refrigerate the cream cheese for 2 hours.
6. Serve.

Serving Suggestion: Serve the cherry dessert with fresh berries on top.

Variation Tip: Add vanilla extracts to the dessert.

Nutritional Information Per Serving:

Calories 153 | Fat 1g |Sodium 8mg | Carbs 66g | Fiber 0.8g | Sugar 56g | Protein 1g

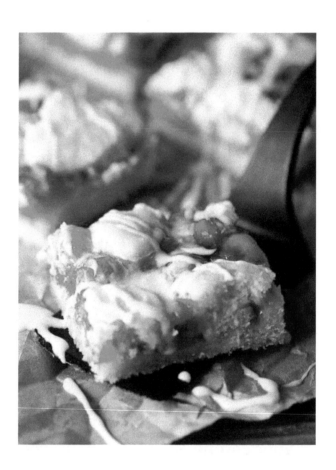

Vanilla Pudding

Prep Time: 15 minutes.

Cook Time: 8 minutes.

Serves: 4

Ingredients:

- 2 cups of milk
- 1/4 teaspoon salt
- 1/2 cup milk
- 3 tablespoons cornstarch
- 3/4 teaspoons pure vanilla extract
- 1/8 teaspoons stevia
- 2 teaspoons buttery spread

Preparation:

1. Warm 2 cup milk in a saucepan.
2. Mix cornstarch with ½ cup milk in a bowl and pour into the saucepan.
3. Cook this milk mixture for 3 minutes until it thickens,
4. Stir in remaining ingredients, then mix well.
5. Allow this pudding to cool and serve.

Serving Suggestion: Serve the pudding with chocolate syrup or berries on top.

Variation Tip: Add crushed walnuts or pecans to the custard.

Nutritional Information Per Serving:

Calories 198 | Fat 14g |Sodium 272mg | Carbs 34g | Fiber 1g | Sugar 9.3g | Protein 1.3g

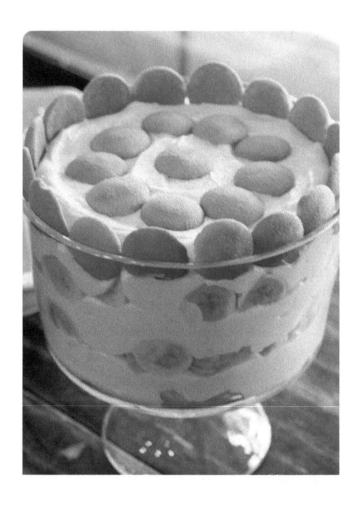

Banana Cookies

Prep Time: 10 minutes.

Cook Time: 15 minutes.

Serves: 4

Ingredients:

- 2 ripe bananas
- 1/3 cup almond milk
- 1 cup all-purpose flour
- 1/2 teaspoon baking powder

Preparation:

1. At 350 degrees F, preheat your oven.
2. Mash bananas with almond milk in a mixing bowl.
3. Stir in baking powder and flour, then mix well.
4. Divide the batter into 13 cookies using a scoop onto a baking sheet with parchment paper.
5. Bake these cookies for 15 minutes in the oven.
6. Allow the cookies to cool.
7. Serve.

Serving Suggestion: Serve the cookies with chocolate sauce.

Variation Tip: Roll the cookies in crushed nuts or coconut flakes before cooking.

Nutritional Information Per Serving:

Calories 159 | Fat 3g |Sodium 277mg | Carbs 21g | Fiber 1g | Sugar 9g | Protein 2g

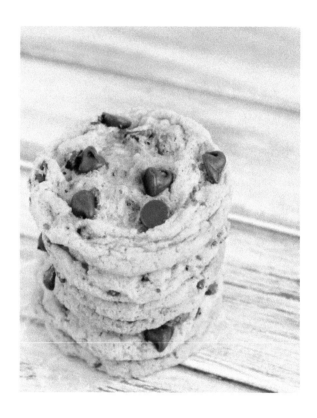

Sweet Potato Cheesecake

Prep Time: 10 minutes.

Cook Time: 15 minutes.

Serves: 6

Ingredients:

- 1 egg, whole
- ¼ cup yogurt cheese
- 1/2 cup coconut milk
- 1/8 teaspoons pumpkin pie spice
- ½ teaspoons vanilla
- 1 tablespoon maple syrup
- 2 package Lean & Green honey sweet potatoes
- ½ teaspoons sweet leaf stevia powdered

To garnish:

- 15 almonds, chopped

Preparation:

1. Blend honey sweet potato fueling with the rest of the ingredients in a bowl.
2. Divide this mixture into 6 muffin cups and drizzle almond on top.
3. Bake for 15 in the oven at 350 degrees F.
4. Serve.

Serving Suggestion: Serve the cakes with cream frosting on top.

Variation Tip: Add chocolate chips or a teaspoon of crushed nuts to the batter for the change of flavor.

Nutritional Information Per Serving:

Calories 245 | Fat 14g |Sodium 122mg | Carbs 23.3g | Fiber 1.2g | Sugar 12g | Protein 4.3g

Cauliflower Breakfast Casserole

Prep Time: 10 minutes.

Cook Time: 55 minutes.

Serves: 8

Ingredients:

- 8 ounces turkey sausage, cooked
- ¼ cup onion, chopped
- 2 cups cauliflower florets
- ½ teaspoon Jalapeno Seasoning
- ¼ teaspoon salt
- ¼ teaspoon black pepper
- 6 turkey bacon slices, cooked and chopped
- 2 cups Mexican cheese, shredded
- 8 large eggs
- 16 ounces egg whites
- ¼ cup almond milk

Preparation:

1. At 350 degrees F, preheat your oven.
2. Grease a baking dish with cooking spray.
3. Saute turkey sausage in a skillet until golden brown.
4. Saute onions and cauliflower in a same skillet until golden.

5. Stir in black pepper, salt, jalapeno seasoning then mix well.
6. Sread the cauliflower mixture in the prepared baking dish.
7. Top this mixture with cheese and bacon.
8. Beat egg whites with eggs and almond milk in a bowl.
9. Pour this mixture over the turkey mixture.
10. Bake for 45 minutes in the oven.
11. Garnish with green onions.
12. Serve warm.

Serving Suggestion: Enjoy this breakfast casserole with a refreshing smoothie.

Variation Tip: Add some chopped or shredded zucchini to the casserole.

Nutritional Information Per Serving:

Calories 244 | Fat 7.9g |Sodium 704mg | Carbs 19g | Fiber 2g | Sugar 14g | Protein 14g

Quinoa Pudding

Prep Time: 10 minutes.

Cook Time: 25 minutes.

Serves: 4

Ingredients:

- 1 cup quinoa
- 4 cups coconut milk
- 1/3 cup maple syrup
- 1 ½ teaspoons vanilla extract
- 1 teaspoon cinnamon
- 1/4 teaspoon salt

Preparation:

1. Mix quinoa, milk, maple, vanilla, cinnamon and salt in a saucepan.
2. Boil this mixture, reduce the heat and cook for 25 minutes.
3. Garnish with your favorite toppings.
4. Serve warm.

Serving Suggestion: Serve this pudding with toasted bread slices.

Variation Tip: Add chopped berries and nuts to the pudding.

Nutritional Information Per Serving:

Calories 214 | Fat 5.1g |Sodium 231mg | Carbs 31g | Fiber 5g | Sugar 2.1g | Protein 7g

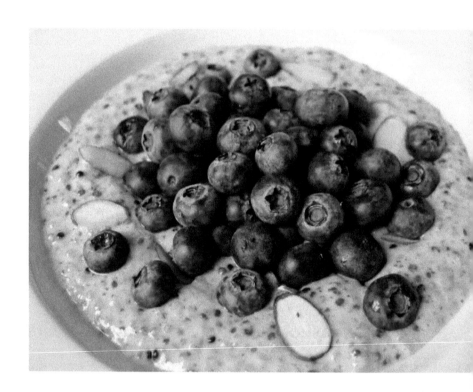

Cranberry Sweet Potato Muffins

Prep Time: 15 minutes.

Cook Time: 20 minutes.

Serves: 4

Ingredients:

- 2 tablespoons butter, melted
- 1/4 cup brown sugar
- 1 egg
- 1 teaspoon vanilla
- 1/4 cup skim milk
- 1/2 cup curd cottage cheese
- 1/2 cup cooked sweet potato, mashed
- 3/4 cup white whole wheat flour
- 1 teaspoon baking powder
- 1 cup fresh cranberries

Preparation:

1. Mix all the ingredients for batter in a bowl until smooth.
2. Stir in cranberries then divide the batter into muffin cups.
3. Bake for 20 minutes at 350 degrees F.
4. Allow the cranberries to cool then serve.

Serving Suggestion: Enjoy these muffins with a refreshing smoothie.

Variation Tip: Add some riasins to the muffins.

Nutritional Information Per Serving:

Calories 225 | Fat 9g |Sodium 118mg | Carbs 35.4g | Fiber 2.9g | Sugar 15g | Protein 6.5g

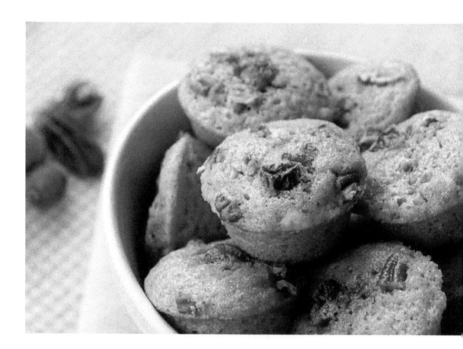

Quinoa Bars

Prep Time: 15 minutes.

Cook Time: 20 minutes.

Serves: 6

Ingredients:

- 1 cup whole wheat flour
- 1 ½ cup cooked quinoa
- 2 cup oats
- 1/2 cup nuts, chopped
- 1 teaspoon cinnamon
- 1 teaspoon baking soda
- 2 tablespoons chia seeds
- 2/3 cup peanut butter
- 1/2 cup honey
- 2 eggs
- 2/3 cup applesauce
- 1teaspoons vanilla
- 1/2 teaspoon salt
- 1/3 cup craisins
- 1/3 cup chocolate chips

Preparation:

1. Mix quinoa with honey, peanut butter, eggs, vanilla, applesauce in a small bowl.
2. Stir in rest of the ingredients then mix well.

3. Spread this mixture in a 9x13 greased baking dish.

4. Bake for 20 minutes at 375 degrees F then cut into bars.

5. Serve.

Serving Suggestion: Enjoy these bars with a strawberry smoothie.

Variation Tip: Add some goji berries to the bars.

Nutritional Information Per Serving:

Calories 163 | Fat 2.5g |Sodium 15.6mg | Carbs 49.5g | Fiber 7.6g | Sugar 28g | Protein 3.5g

Buckwheat Crepes

Prep Time: 15 minutes.

Cook Time: 10 minutes.

Serves: 4

Ingredients:

- 2/3 cup buckwheat flour
- 1/3 cup whole wheat flour
- 2 eggs
- 1 ¼ cup skim milk
- 1 tablespoon honey
- Fruit and Greek yogurt, for filling

Preparation:

1. Mix flours with eggs, milk, and honey in a bowl until smooth.
2. Set a nonstick skillet over medium heat.
3. Add a ¼ cup batter into the skillet, spread it evenly then cook for 2 minutes per side.
4. Transfer the crepe to a plate and then cook the remaining batter in the same way.
5. Garnish with fruits and yogurt.
6. Serve.

Serving Suggestion: Enjoy these crepes with a blueberry smoothie.

Variation Tip: Add some blueberries to the crepes filling.

Nutritional Information Per Serving:

Calories 112 | Fat 25g |Sodium 132mg | Carbs 44g | Fiber 3.9g | Sugar 3g | Protein 8.9g

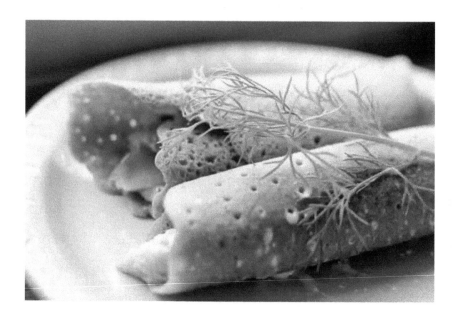

Oatmeal Pancakes

Prep Time: 10 minutes.

Cook Time: 10 minutes.

Serves: 6

Ingredients:

- 2/3 cup Greek Yogurt
- 3 tablespoons skim milk
- 1 tablespoon applesauce
- 1 egg
- 1/2 cup white whole wheat flour
- 3/4 cup oats, crushed
- 1 teaspoon baking powder
- 1/2 teaspoon baking soda
- 1 tablespoon ground flaxseed
- 1 teaspoon cinnamon

Preparation:

1. Mix flours and rest of the ingredients in a bowl until smooth.
2. Set a hot griddle over medium heat.

3. Pour a ladle of battter over the griddle and cook the pancake for 2 mintues per side.
4. Transfer to a plate and cook remaining pancakes in the same manner.
5. Serve warm.

Serving Suggestion: Enjoy these pancakes with a spinach smoothie.

Variation Tip: Add chopped nuts to the batter.

Nutritional Information Per Serving:

Calories 190 | Fat 15g |Sodium 595mg | Carbs 11g | Fiber 3g | Sugar 12g | Protein 9g

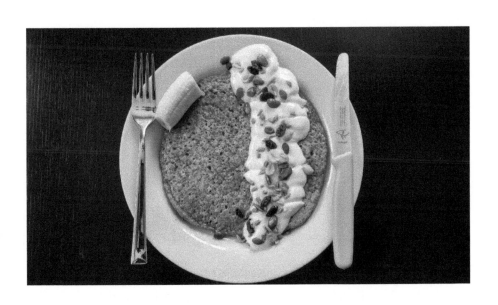

Blueberry Muffins

Prep Time: 15 minutes.

Cook Time: 30 minutes.

Serves: 4

Ingredients:

- 2 tablespoons butter, melted
- 1 cup fresh blueberries
- 1/4 cup sugar
- 1 egg
- 1 teaspoon vanilla
- 1/4 cup skim milk
- 1/2 cup curd cottage cheese
- 1/2 cup cooked sweet potato, mashed
- 3/4 cup whole wheat flour
- 1 teaspoon baking powder

Preparation:

1. Mix sweet potato mash with all the ingredients except cranberries in a bowl until smooth.
2. Fold in blueberries then mix evenly.
3. Divide the batter into the muffin tray and bake for 30 minutes at 350 degrees F.

4. Serve.

Serving Suggestion: Enjoy these muffins with a strawberry smoothie.

Variation Tip : Add raisins to the muffin batter.

Nutritional Information Per Serving:

Calories 197 | Fat 15g |Sodium 202mg | Carbs 58.5g | Fiber 4g | Sugar 1g | Protein 7.3g

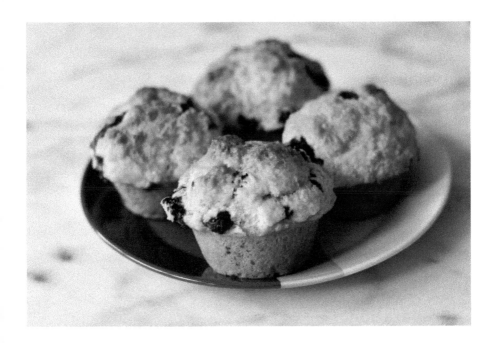

Berry Quinoa

Prep Time: 10 minutes.

Cook Time: 20 minutes.

Serves: 4

Ingredients:

- ¼ cup quinoa, rinsed
- 1/2 cup almond milk
- 1/2 cup berries
- 1 dash cinnamon
- 1/2 teaspoon vanilla

Toppings

- Nuts
- Fruit
- Chocolate chips
- Nut butter
- Agave/honey

Preparation:

1. Mix quinoa with milk, vanilla, cinnamon and berries in a saucepan.

2. Cook to a boil, reduce its heat and cook for 20 minutes until liquid is absorved.
3. Garnish with desired toppings.
4. Serve.

Serving Suggestion: Enjoy this quinoa with a cranberry muffin.

Variation Tip: Add roasted nuts to the quinoa.

Nutritional Information Per Serving:
Calories 163 | Fat 6.5g |Sodium 548mg | Carbs 3.4g | Fiber 2g | Sugar 1g | Protein 2g

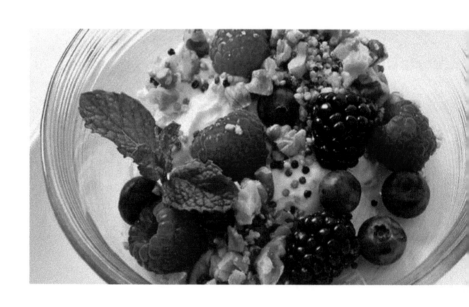

Celery Salad

Prep Time: 5 minutes.

Cook Time: 0 minutes.

Serves: 2

Ingredients:

- 1 cup celery, chopped
- 1 tablespoon mint, chopped
- 1 teaspoon lemon juice
- 1 teaspoon olive oil

Preparation:

1. Mix celery with mint, lemon juice and olive oil in a salad bowl.
2. Serve.

Serving Suggestion: Serve this salad with grilled shrimp.

Variation Tip: Drizzle dried herbs and cumin on top.

Nutritional Information Per Serving:

Calories 148 | Fat 22g |Sodium 350mg | Carbs 32.2g | Fiber 0.7g | Sugar 1g | Protein 4.3g

Taco Salad

-Prep Time: 5 minutes.

Cook Time: 0 minutes.

Serves: 2

Ingredients:

- 5 ounces ground turkey
- 1 tablespoon taco seasoning
- 2 tablespoons salsa
- 1 cup romaine lettuce
- 1 cup iceberg lettuce
- 1/2 cup diced tomatoes
- 1 tablespoon water

Preparation:

1. Saute turkey with taco seasoning in a skillet until golden brown.
2. Transfer to a salad bowl and stir in salsa, lettuces, tomatoes and water.
3. Mix well and serve.

Serving Suggestion: Serve this salad with grilled chicken.

Variation Tip: Drizzle black pepper ground on top before serving.

Nutritional Information Per Serving:

Calories 345 | Fat 9g |Sodium 48mg | Carbs 14g | Fiber 1g | Sugar 2g | Protein 20g

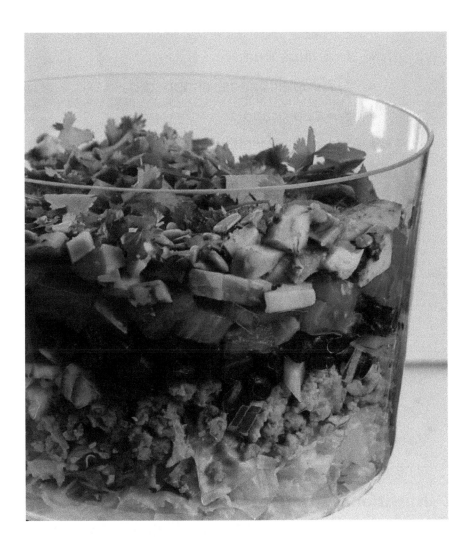

Yogurt Trail Mix Bars

Prep Time: 15 minutes.

Cook Time: 0 minutes.

Serves: 4

Ingredients:

- 2 cups Greek yogurt
- 1 ½ cups fruit
- 1/2 cup almonds, chopped
- 3/4 cup granola
- 1/4 cup chocolate chips

Preparation:

1. Mix yogurt with fruit, almonds, granola and chocolate chips in a bowl.
2. Spread this mixture in a shallow tray and freeze for 1 hour.
3. Cut the mixture into bars.
4. Serve.

Serving Suggestion: Serve these bars with a berry compote.

Variation Tip: Pour melted chocolates on top and then slice to serve.

Nutritional Information Per Serving:

Calories 204 | Fat 3g |Sodium 216mg | Carbs 17g | Fiber 3g | Sugar 4g | Protein 11g

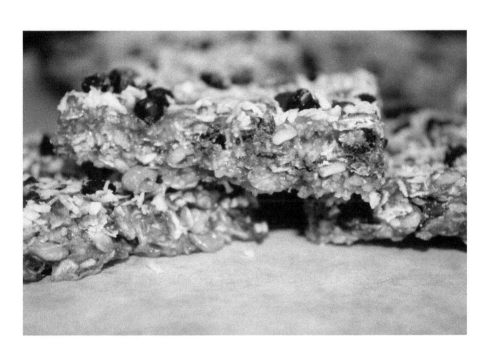

Curried Tuna Salad

Prep Time: 15 minutes.

Cook Time: 0 minutes.

Serves: 2

Ingredients:

- 2 cans of tuna, drained
- ¼ cup hummus
- ¼ cup avocado, smashed
- ½ cup apple, chopped
- ¼ cup onion, diced
- 1 tablespoon lemon juice
- 2 teaspoons curry powder
- 1/2 teaspoon dry mustard powder

Preparation:

1. Mix tuna with rest of the ingredients in a salad bowl.
2. Serve fresh.

Serving Suggestion: Serve this salad with grilled shrimp.

Variation Tip: Drizzle shredded coconut on top before serving.

Nutritional Information Per Serving:

Calories 280 | Fat 9g |Sodium 318mg | Carbs 19g | Fiber 5g | Sugar 3g | Protein 17g

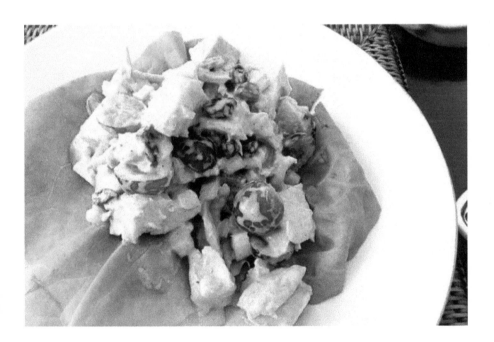

Tuna Quinoa Cakes

Prep Time: 15 minutes.

Cook Time: 20 minutes.

Serves: 4

Ingredients:

- 1/2 cup cooked sweet potato, mashed
- 2 cans tuna, drained
- 3/4 cup cooked quinoa
- 1/4 cup green onion, chopped
- 2 garlic cloves, minced
- 1 tablespoon lemon juice
- 1 egg
- 1/4 cup plain yogurt
- 1 tablespoon mustard
- 1/2 teaspoon cayenne pepper
- 1 teaspoon paprika
- 1/2 cup breadcrumbs

Preparation:

1. In a small bowl, combine the tuna and sweet potato and mix well.
2. Add remaining ingredients and stir until well combined.
3. Make 6 patties out of this mixture.

4. Place the patties in a greased baking sheet and bake for 20 minutes at 400 degrees F.
5. Flip the patties once cooked half way through.
6. Serve warm.

Serving Suggestion: Serve the cakes with cream cheese dip on the side.

Variation Tip: Add shredded parmesan before cooking.

Nutritional Information Per Serving:
Calories 273 | Fat 8g |Sodium 146mg | Carbs 18g | Fiber 5g | Sugar 1g | Protein 7g

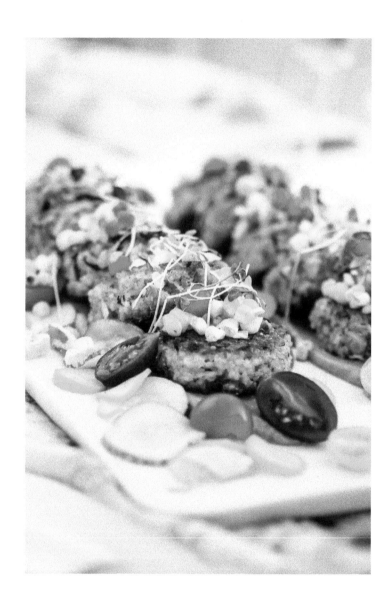

Taco Cups

Prep Time: 15 minutes.

Cook Time: 25 minutes.

Serves: 4

Ingredients:

- 2 Sargento cheese slices
- 4 ounces lean ground beef
- 1 teaspoon taco seasoning

Toppings:

- Lettuce and tomatoes
- 1 tablespoon sour cream

Preparation:

1. At 375 degrees F, preheat your oven.
2. Sauté beef in a skillet for 5 minutes.
3. Stir in taco seasoning then mix well.
4. Layer a baking sheet with wax paper.
5. Place cheese slices in the baking sheet and bake for 7 minutes in the oven.
6. Allow the cheese to cool and then place each cheese round in the muffin tray.
7. Press the cheese into cups and divide the beef into these cups.

8. Garnish with desired toppings.

9. Serve warm.

Serving Suggestion: Serve the cups with guacamole.

Variation Tip: Add shredded cheese to the filling.

Nutritional Information Per Serving:

Calories 240 | Fat 25g |Sodium 244mg | Carbs 16g | Fiber 1g | Sugar 1g | Protein 27g

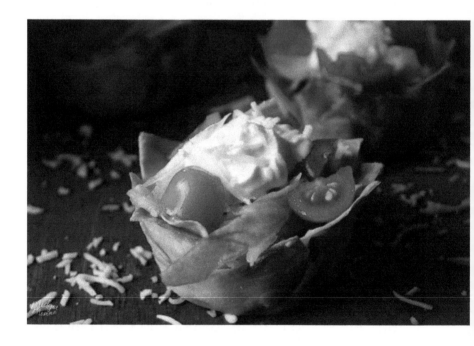

Caprese Spaghetti Squash Nests

Prep Time: 15 minutes.

Cook Time: 1 hr 35 minutes.

Serves: 4

Ingredients:

For the Nests:

- 1 medium spaghetti squash
- 1/4 teaspoon salt
- 1/4 teaspoon black pepper
- 1/4 teaspoon garlic powder
- 3 tablespoons egg whites

Filling:

- 1 cup cherry tomatoes
- 1/4 teaspoon salt
- 1/4 teaspoon black pepper
- 4 ounces mozzarella cheese, shredded
- 1/4 cup basil, chopped

Preparation:

1. At 375 degrees F, preheat your oven.
2. Cut the spaghetti squash in half and place in the baking sheet.
3. Bake the squash for 45 minutes in the oven.
4. Scrape the squash with a fork and divide the shreds in the muffin tray.

5. Beat egg whites with garlic powder, black pepper and salt.
6. Divide this liquid mixture into the muffin cups, make a nest at the center of each and bake for 20 minutes.
7. Spread tomatoes in a baking sheet and bake for 20 minutes in the oven.
8. Divide the roasted tomaotes in the spaghetti squash and top them with cheese and rest of the ingredients.
9. Bake for 10 minutes in the oven.
10. Serve warm.

Serving Suggestion: Serve the nests with spinach or cream cheese dip.

Variation Tip: Add shredded parmesan on top.

Nutritional Information Per Serving:

Calories 282 | Fat 4g |Sodium 232mg | Carbs 7g | Fiber 1g | Sugar 0g | Protein 14g

Fire Cracker Shrimp

Prep Time: 15 minutes.

Cook Time: 6 minutes.

Serves: 4

Ingredients:

- 11 ounces raw shrimp, peeled
- 2 tablespoons Apricot Preserves
- 1 teaspoon lite soy sauce
- ½ teaspoon sriracha sauce
- 1 teaspoon sesame oil

Preparation:

1. Place apricot in a small bowl and heat for 20 seconds in the microwave.
2. Mix oil, sriracha sauce, soy sauce and apricot mixture in a bowl.
3. Thread the shrimp on the wooden skewers and brush them with apricot mixture.
4. Grill these skewers for 3 minutes per side.
5. Serve warm.

Serving Suggestion: Serve the shrimp with zucchini fries.

Variation Tip: Add crumbled cheese on top.

Nutritional Information Per Serving:

Calories 229 | Fat 5g |Sodium 510mg | Carbs 37g | Fiber 5g | Sugar 4g | Protein 21g

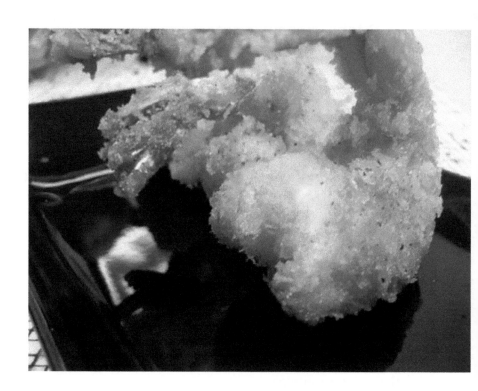

Crispy Zucchini Chips

Prep Time: 15 minutes.

Cook Time: 4 hrs.

Serves: 4

Ingredients:

- 1 ½ cups zucchini
- 1 teaspoon olive oil
- 1/8 teaspoons salt

Preparation:

1. At 200 degrees F, preheat your oven.
2. Layer a baking sheet with wax paper and grease with cooking spray.
3. Spread the zucchini slices in the baking sheet and bake for 4 hours.
4. Flip the zucchinin once cooked half way through.
5. Serve warm.

Serving Suggestion: Serve the chips with tomato sauce.

Variation Tip: Drizzle black pepper on top before serving.

Nutritional Information Per Serving:

Calories 101 | Fat 7g |Sodium 269mg | Carbs 5g | Fiber 4g | Sugar 12g | Protein 1g

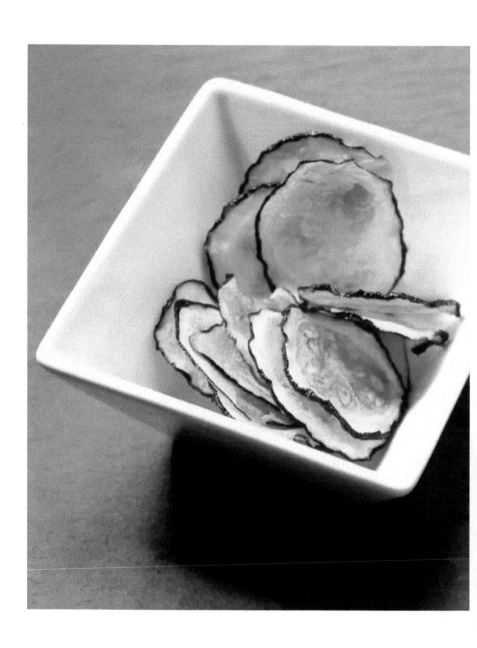

Baked Kale Chips

Prep Time: 15 minutes.

Cook Time: 15 minutes.

Serves: 4

Ingredients:

- 4 ½ cups kale
- 1 tablespoon olive oil
- 1/4 teaspoon salt

Preparation:

1. At 450-degree F, preheat your oven.
2. Layer a baking sheet with parchment paper.
3. Toss the kale leaves with salt, and olive oil in the baking sheet.
4. Spread them evenly then bake for 15 minutes in the oven.
5. Serve.

Serving Suggestion: Serve these chips with chilli garlic sauce.

Variation Tip: Add some paprika or red pepper flakes to the topping.

Nutritional Information Per Serving:

Calories 118 | Fat 11g |Sodium 110mg | Carbs 4g | Fiber 5g | Sugar 3g | Protein 1g

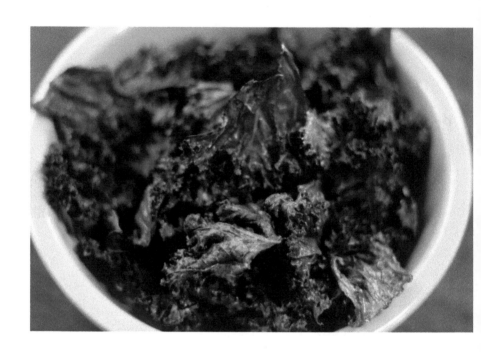

Chia Seed Pudding

Prep Time: 15 minutes.

Cook Time: 0 minute.

Serves: 2

Ingredients:

- 2 cups almond milk
- 1/2 cup chia seeds
- 1/4 cup almond butter
- 1/4 cup cocoa powder unsweetened
- 4 dates large, pitted and chopped
- 1 teaspoon pure vanilla extract

Preparation:

1. Blend all the pudding ingredients in a bowl.
2. Cover and refrigerate this pudding for 4 hours.
3. Serve.

Serving Suggestion: Serve the pudding with goji berries on top.

Variation Tip: Add white chocolate syrup on top.

Nutritional Information Per Serving:

Calories 361 | Fat 10g |Sodium 218mg | Carbs 56g | Fiber 10g | Sugar 30g | Protein 4g

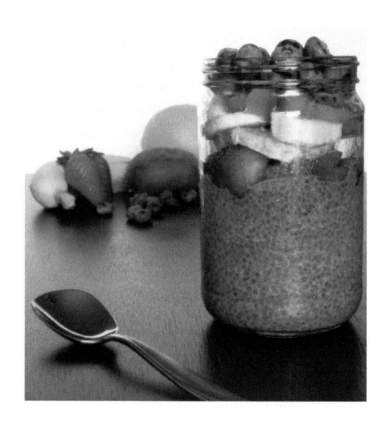

Grilled Buffalo Shrimp

Prep Time: 15 minutes.

Cook Time: 8 minutes.

Serves: 4

Ingredients:

- 11 ounce raw shrimp, peeled
- 1/4 cup Frank's Hot Sauce
- 1 tablespoon butter

Preparation:

1. Mix butter with hot sauce in a bowl.
2. Thread the shrimp on the skewers and brush them with butter mixture.
3. Grill these skewers for 2 minutes per side while basting with butter sauce.
4. Serve warm.

Serving Suggestion: Serve the shrimps with tomato ketchup.

Variation Tip: Coat the shrimp in breadcrumbs before cooking.

Nutritional Information Per Serving:

Calories 275 | Fat 16g |Sodium 255mg | Carbs 1g | Fiber 1.2g | Sugar 5g | Protein 19g

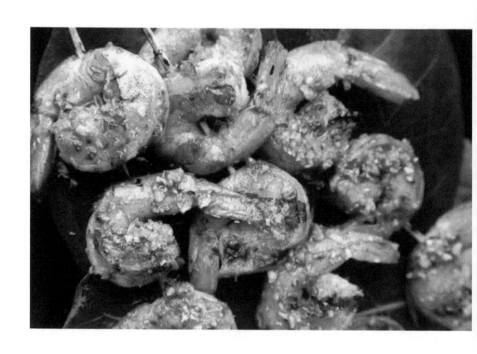

Strawberry Ice Cream

Prep Time: 10 minutes.

Cook Time: 0 minutes.

Serves: 6

Ingredients:

- 16 ounce strawberries, frozen
- 3/4 cup Greek yogurt plain
- 2 tablespoons balsamic vinegar
- 2 tablespoons honey

Preparation:

1. Blend all the ingredients for ice cream in a blender until smooth.
2. Divide the mixture in the ice-cream molds.
3. Freeze the ice cream for 4 hours.
4. Serve.

Serving Suggestion: Serve the ice cream with fresh berries on top.

Variation Tip: Add strawberry preserves on top of the ice cream.

Nutritional Information Per Serving:

Calories 118 | Fat 20g |Sodium 192mg | Carbs 23.7g | Fiber 0.9g | Sugar 19g | Protein 5.2g

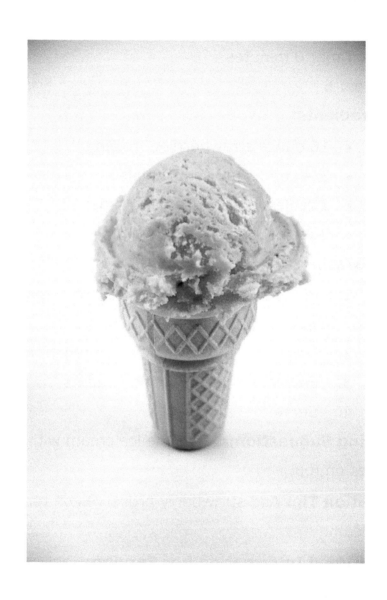

Strawberry Yogurt

Prep Time: 5 minutes.

Cook Time: 0 minutes.

Serves: 2

Ingredients:

Spices

- 1 cup Greek yogurt plain
- 3/4 cup strawberry fruit spread

Preparation:

1. Blend yogurt with strawberries in a blender.
2. Serve.

Serving Suggestion: Serve the yogurt with berries on top.

Variation Tip: Add chopped pecans to the yogurt as well.

Nutritional Information Per Serving:

Calories 248 | Fat 16g |Sodium 95mg | Carbs 38.4g | Fiber 0.3g | Sugar 10g | Protein 14.1g

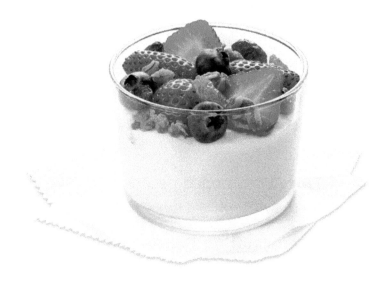

Banana Pops

Prep Time: 15 minutes.

Cook Time: 0 minutes.

Serves: 2

Ingredients:

- 3 bananas
- 3 tablespoons cacao powder raw
- 2 liquid stevia drops
- 3 ounces water
- 1/4 cup cacao nibs raw
- 1/4 cup goji berries raw

Preparation:

1. Insert a stick into each banana.
2. Place these bananas in the freezer for 30 minutes.
3. Mash the remaining banana with stevia, water and cacao powder in a bowl.
4. Dip the bananas on the stick in the cacao mmixture.
5. Coat them with cacao nibs and gji berries.
6. Serve.

Serving Suggestion: Serve the pops with chocolate or apple sauce.

Variation Tip: Dip the bananas in white chocolate syrup.

Nutritional Information Per Serving:

Calories 117 | Fat 12g |Sodium 79mg | Carbs 24.8g | Fiber 1.1g | Sugar 18g | Protein 5g

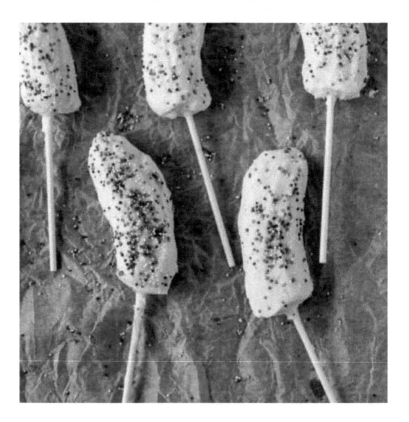

Lean and Green Smoothie

Prep Time: 5 minutes.

Cook Time: 0 minutes.

Serves: 2

Ingredients:

- 2 ½ cups kale leaves, stemmed
- 1 cup pineapple, cubed
- ¾ cup apple juice, chilled
- ½ cup seedless green grapes, frozen
- ½ cup Granny Smith apple, chopped
- 1 cup green grapes, halved

Preparation:

1. Blend kale with grapes with apple and pineapple in a blender.
2. Serve with halved grapes.
3. Enjoy.

Serving Suggestion: Enjoy this smoothie with breakfast muffins.

Variation Tip: Add some strawberries to the smoothie.

Nutritional Information Per Serving:

Calories 84 | Fat 7.9g |Sodium 704mg | Carbs 19g | Fiber 2g | Sugar 14g | Protein 1g

Medifast Patties

Prep Time: 10 minutes.

Cook Time: 20 minutes.

Serves: 4

Ingredients:

- 1 3/4 lbs. Dungeness crab meat
- 1 tablespoon red bell pepper, diced
- 1 tablespoon green bell pepper, diced
- 1 tablespoon parsley leaves, chopped
- 1 ½ tablespoon heavy mayonnaise
- 2 eggs 3 teaspoons baking powder
- 1 teaspoon Worcestershire sauce
- 1 teaspoon Old Bay seasoning
- 10 cooking spray

Preparation:

1. Mix crab meat with bell peppers, parsley, mayonnaise, baking powder, Worcestershire sauce and old bay seasoning in a bowl.
2. Make small patties out of this mixture.
3. Set a skillet, greased with cooking spray, over medium heat.
4. Sear the patties for 5 minutes per side.

5. Enjoy.

Serving Suggestion: Serve these patties with toasted bread slices.

Variation Tip: Add chopped carrots and broccoli to the cakes.

Nutritional Information Per Serving:

Calories 214 | Fat 5.1g |Sodium 231mg | Carbs 31g | Fiber 5g | Sugar 2.1g | Protein 17g

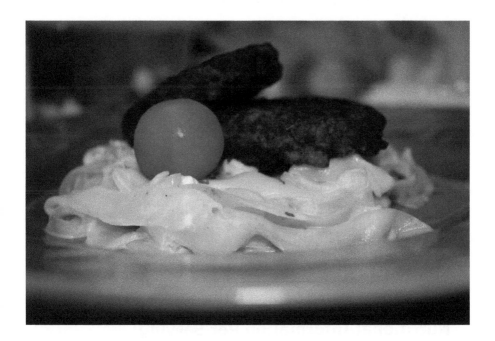

Green Colada Smoothie

Prep Time: 5 minutes.

Cook Time: 0 minutes.

Serves: 2

Ingredients:

- 1 cup Greek yogurt
- 1 cup frozen pineapple
- 1 cup baby spinach
- ½ cup lite coconut milk
- ½ teaspoon vanilla extract
- Coconut flakes for garnish

Preparation:

1. Blend yogurt with pineapple, spinach, coconut milk, and vanilla in a blender until smooth.
2. Garnish with coconut flakes and serve.

Serving Suggestion: Enjoy this smoothie with breakfast muffins.

Variation Tip: Add some strawberries to the smoothie.

Nutritional Information Per Serving:

Calories 325 | Fat 9g |Sodium 118mg | Carbs 35.4g | Fiber 2.9g | Sugar 15g | Protein 26.5g

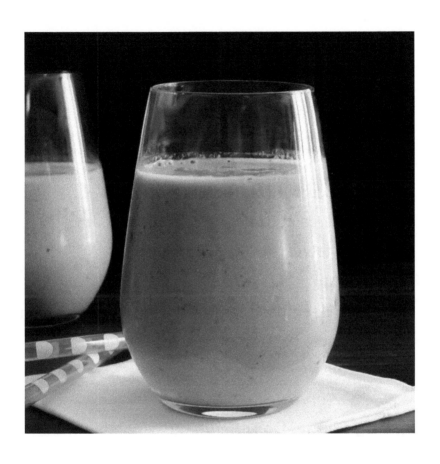

Green Apple Smoothie

Prep Time: 5 minutes.

Cook Time: 0 minutes.

Serves: 2

Ingredients:

- 2 ripe bananas
- 1 ripe pear, peeled, chopped
- 2 cups kale leaves, chopped
- ½ cup of orange juice
- ½ cup of cold water
- 12 ice cubes
- 1 tablespoon ground flaxseed

Preparation:

1. Blend bananas with pear, kale leaves, orange juice, cold water, ice cubes and flaxseed in a blender.
2. Serve.

Serving Suggestion: Serve this smoothie with morning muffins.

Variation Tip: Add some strawberries to the smoothie.

Nutritional Information Per Serving:

Calories 213 | Fat 2.5g |Sodium 15.6mg | Carbs 49.5g | Fiber 7.6g | Sugar 28g | Protein 3.5g

Spinach Smoothie

Prep Time: 5 minutes.

Cook Time: 0 minutes.

Serves: 2

Ingredients:

- 1 cup fresh spinach
- 1 banana
- ½ green apple
- 4 hulled strawberries
- 4 (1 inch) pieces frozen mango
- ⅓ cup whole milk
- 1 scoop vanilla protein powder
- 1 teaspoon honey

Preparation:

1. Blend spinach with banana with the green apple with strawberries, mango, milk, protein powder and honey in a blender.
2. Serve.

Serving Suggestion: Enjoy this smoothie with breakfast muffins.

Variation Tip: Add some blueberries to the smoothie.

Nutritional Information Per Serving:

Calories 312 | Fat 25g |Sodium 132mg | Carbs 44g | Fiber 3.9g | Sugar 3g | Protein 18.9g

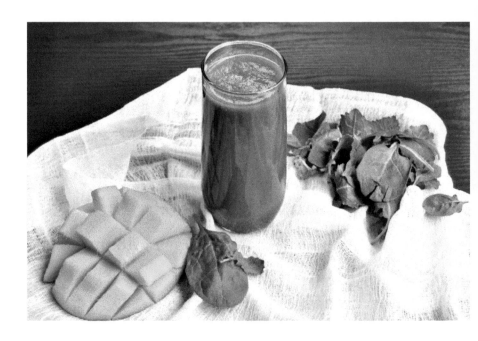

Kale and Cheese Muffins

Prep Time: 10 minutes.

Cook Time: 25 minutes.

Serves: 9

Ingredients:

- 9 large eggs
- 1 cup liquid egg whites
- 3/4 cup plain Greek yogurt
- 2 ounces goat cheese crumbled
- 1/2 teaspoon salt
- 10 ounces kale
- 2 cups cherry tomatoes
- cooking spray

Preparation:

1. At 375 degrees F, preheat your oven.
2. Beat eggs with goat cheese, yogurt, and egg whites in a bowl.
3. Stir in cherry tomatoes and kale, then divide this mixture into a muffin tray.
4. Bake the muffin cups for 25 minutes in the preheated oven.
5. Enjoy.

Serving Suggestion: Serve these muffins with a green smoothie.

Variation Tip: Add chopped nuts to the batter.

Nutritional Information Per Serving:

Calories 290 | Fat 15g |Sodium 595mg | Carbs 11g | Fiber 3g | Sugar 12g | Protein 29g

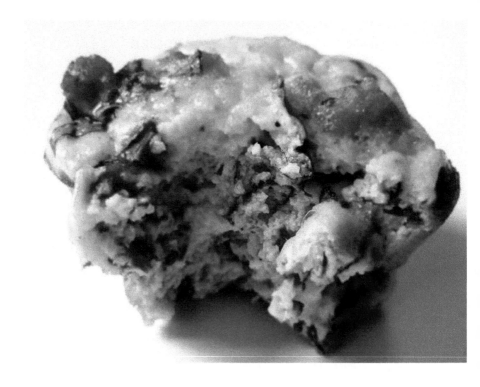

Matcha Avocado Smoothie

Prep Time: 5 minutes.

Cook Time: 0 minutes.

Serves: 2

Ingredients:

- 1/2 avocado, peeled and cubed
- 1/3 cucumber
- 2 cups spinach
- 6 ounces coconut milk
- 6 ounces almond milk
- 1 teaspoon matcha powder
- 1/2 lime juice
- 1/2 scoop vanilla protein powder
- 1/2 teaspoon chia seeds

Preparation:

1. Blend avocado flesh with cucumber and the rest of the ingredients in a blender until smooth.
2. Serve.

Serving Suggestion: Enjoy this smoothie with breakfast muffins.

Variation Tip : Add some strawberries to the smoothie.

Nutritional Information Per Serving:

Calories 297 | Fat 15g |Sodium 202mg | Carbs 58.5g |
Fiber 4g | Sugar 1g | Protein 7.3g

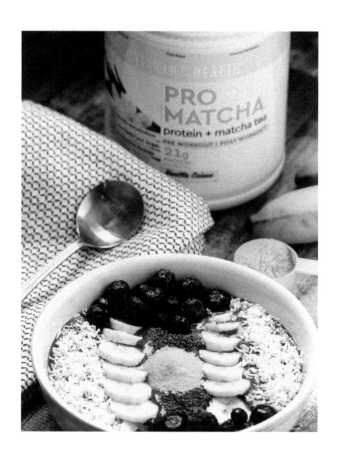

Egg Cups

Prep Time: 10 minutes.

Cook Time: 13 minutes.

Serves: 4

Ingredients:

- 4 eggs
- 8 egg whites
- ¼ c chopped green chilies
- 1 bunch green onions chopped
- 12 pieces of Canadian bacon
- 1 cup ripped spinach
- 1/8 teaspoons salt
- ½ teaspoons black pepper

Preparation:

1. Beat eggs with egg whites, green chilies, green onions, spinach, black pepper and salt in a bowl.
2. Place a bacon slice in each muffin cup of a muffin tray and press it.
3. Divide the egg mixture into the bacon cup.
4. Bake for 13 minutes in the oven at 350 degrees F.
5. Serve warm.

Serving Suggestion: Serve these cups with a green smoothie.

Variation Tip: Add sautéed ground chicken to the egg filling.

Nutritional Information Per Serving:

Calories 163 | Fat 6.5g |Sodium 548mg | Carbs 3.4g | Fiber 2g | Sugar 1g | Protein 22g

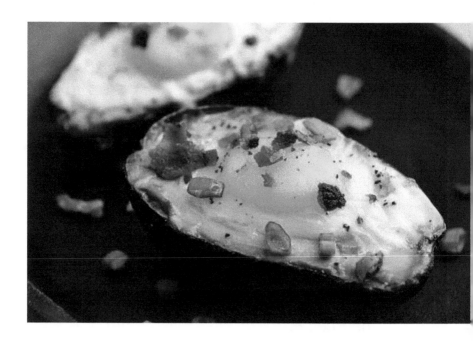

Sweet Potato Rounds

Prep Time: 15 minutes.

Cook Time: 22 minutes.

Serves: 6

Ingredients:

- 2 lbs. sweet potatoes
- 1 ½ tablespoons olive oil
- 1 teaspoon garlic powder
- 1 teaspoon chili powder
- 1 teaspoon salt
- Hot sauce
- Monterrey Jack and cheddar cheese, shredded
- 3 green onions
- Sour cream

Preparation:

1. At 450 degrees F, preheat your oven.
2. Slice the sweet potatoes into ¼ inch thick slices.
3. Toss the slices with 1 teaspoon salt, 1 teaspoon chili powder, 1 teaspoon garlic powder and 1 ½ tablespoon olive oil in a large bowl.
4. Spread these slices in a baking sheet, lined with parchment paper.

5. Bake the sweet potato slices for 10 minutes, flip and bake again for 10 minutes.

6. Top each potato slice with green onions, a dot of hot sauce, and shredded cheese.

7. Bake the potatoes for 2 minutes until the cheese is melted.

8. Garnish with sour cream and serve warm.

Serving Suggestion: Serve these rounds with tomato ketchup or cheese dip.

Variation Tip: Drizzle cinnamon ground on top.

Nutritional Information Per Serving:

Calories 148 | Fat 22g |Sodium 350mg | Carbs 32.2g | Fiber 0.7g | Sugar 1g | Protein 4.3g

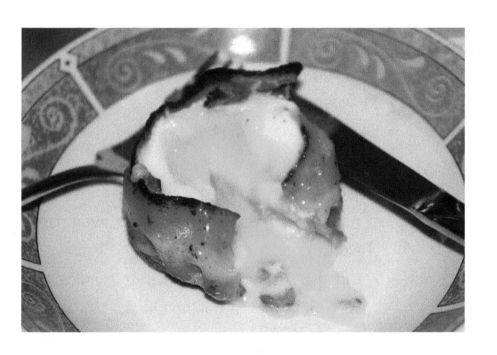

Zucchini Bites

Prep Time: 15 minutes.

Cook Time: 10 minutes.

Serves: 6

Ingredients:

- 2 large zucchinis
- ½ cup pizza sauce
- 1 teaspoon oregano
- 2 cups mozzarella cheese
- ¼ cup parmesan cheese

Preparation:

1. At 450 degrees F, preheat your oven. Layer a baking sheet with a foil sheet.
2. Cut the zucchini into ¼ inch thick slice and place them on the baking sheet.
3. Top each slice with pizza sauce, oregano, and cheese.
4. Bake the zucchini slices for 5-10 minutes until the cheese is melted.
5. Serve warm.

Serving Suggestion: Serve the bites with cheese or yogurt dip.

Variation Tip: Drizzle black pepper ground on top before baking.

Nutritional Information Per Serving:

Calories 145 | Fat 9g |Sodium 48mg | Carbs 4g | Fiber 1g | Sugar 2g | Protein 10g

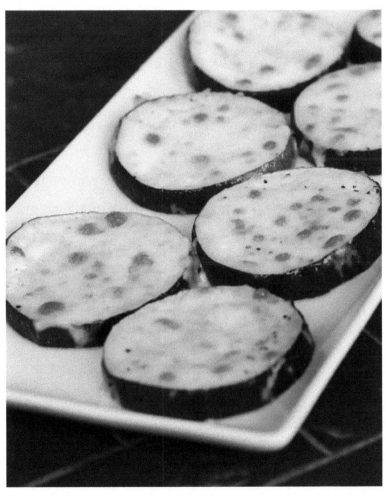

Cauliflower Bites

Prep Time: 15 minutes.

Cook Time: 20 minutes.

Serves: 8

Ingredients:

- 8 cups cauliflower florets
- 2 tablespoons olive oil
- ¼ teaspoon kosher salt
- 2 tablespoons hot sauce
- 1-2 tablespoons Sriracha
- 1 tablespoon butter, melted
- 1 tablespoon lemon juice

Preparation:

1. At 450 degrees F, preheat your oven.
2. Layer a rimmed baking sheet with cooking spray.
3. Toss cauliflower with salt and oil in a large bowl and spread evenly on the baking sheet.
4. Roast the cauliflower florets for 15 minutes in the preheated oven.
5. Mix hot sauce, lemon juice, butter and sriracha in a large bowl.
6. Toss in cauliflower and mix well to coat.

7.   Return the cauliflower to the baking sheet and bake for 5 minutes.

8.   Serve warm.

Serving Suggestion: Serve the cauliflower bites with tomato sauce.

Variation Tip: Coat the cauliflower with breadcrumbs before cooking.

Nutritional Information Per Serving:
Calories 104 | Fat 3g |Sodium 216mg | Carbs 17g | Fiber 3g | Sugar 4g | Protein 1g

Pancetta Wrapped Prunes

Prep Time: 15 minutes.

Cook Time: 11 minutes.

Serves: 8

Ingredients:

- 16 prunes, pitted
- 150g of Gorgonzola
- 16 pancetta slices
- 3 tablespoons vegetable oil
- 3 tablespoons of walnuts
- 1 handful of celery leaves
- Black pepper, to taste

Preparation:

1. Add prunes with water to a cooking pot, cover and boil for 5 minutes then drain.
2. Pat dry the prunes, and remove their pits.
3. Dice the gorgonzola into 16 cubes and insert one cube into each pitted prune.
4. Wrap each prune with a pancetta slice and insert a toothpick to secure it.
5. Set a pan with cooking oil over medium heat and sear the wrapped prunes for 2-3 minutes per side.

6.   Garnish with walnuts, black pepper and celery leaves.

7.   Enjoy.

Serving Suggestion: Serve the rolls with mayonnaise dip.

Variation Tip: Drizzle shredded coconut on top before serving.

Nutritional Information Per Serving:

Calories 180 | Fat 9g |Sodium 318mg | Carbs 19g | Fiber 5g | Sugar 3g | Protein 7g

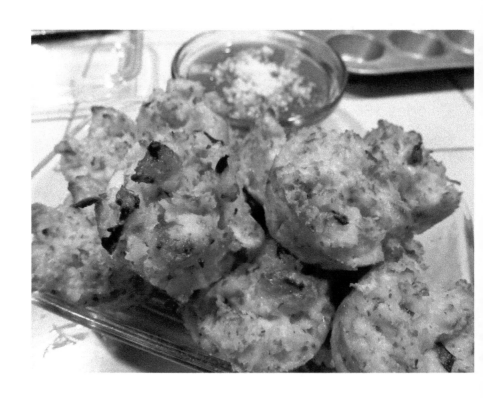

Turkey Lettuce Wraps

Prep Time: 15 minutes.

Cook Time: 8 minutes.

Serves: 6

Ingredients:

- 1 lb. lean ground turkey
- 1 tablespoon vegetable oil
- 1 small onion, diced
- 2 garlic cloves, minced
- 1 teaspoon ginger, grated
- 1 bell pepper, diced
- 1 tablespoon soy sauce
- 2 tablespoons Hoisin
- 1 teaspoon sesame oil
- 2 teaspoons rice vinegar
- 2 green onions, minced
- Salt, to taste
- Black pepper, to taste
- Fresh lettuce leaves

Preparation:

1. Sauté onion with ginger, garlic and cooking oil in a large pan until soft.

2.   Stir in turkey ground and sauté for 3
     minutes.

3.   Add rice vinegar, sesame oil, hoisin and soy
     sauce then mix well.

4.   Stir in green onion and bell peppers then
     sauté for 5 minutes.

5.   Adjust seasoning with black pepper and salt.

6.   Divide this filling into the lettuce leaves.

7.   Serve.

Serving Suggestion: Serve the wraps with cream
cheese dip on the side.

Variation Tip: Toss turkey meat with shredded
parmesan before cooking.

Nutritional Information Per Serving:

Calories 173 | Fat 8g |Sodium 146mg | Carbs 18g |
Fiber 5g | Sugar 1g | Protein 7g

Bell Pepper Bites

Prep Time: 15 minutes.

Cook Time: 4 minutes.

Serves: 9

Ingredients:

- 1 medium green bell pepper
- 1 medium red bell pepper
- 1/4 cup almonds, sliced
- 4 ounces low-fat cream cheese
- 1 teaspoon lemon pepper seasoning blend
- 1 teaspoon lemon juice

Preparation:

1. Slice the peppers in half, lengthwise.
2. Destem and deseed the peppers and cut each half into 6 more pieces.
3. Roast almonds in a skillet for 4 minutes then grind in a food processor.
4. Mix cream cheese with lemon juice and lemon pepper in a mixing bowl for 2 minutes.
5. Stir in the almond ground and mix for 10 seconds.
6. Add this filling to the piping bag and pipe this mixture into the bell pepper piece.
7. Serve.

Serving Suggestion: Serve the peppers with chilli sauce or mayo dip.

Variation Tip: Add shredded cheese to the filling.

Nutritional Information Per Serving:

Calories 140 | Fat 5g |Sodium 244mg | Carbs 16g | Fiber 1g | Sugar 1g | Protein 17g

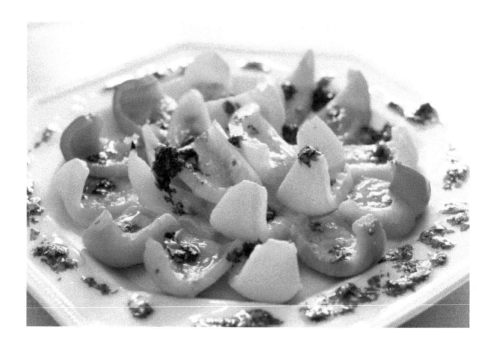

Avocado Shrimp Cucumber

Prep Time: 15 minutes.

Cook Time: 6 minutes.

Serves: 4

Ingredients:

- 1 cucumber, sliced into 1/2-inch slices
- 2 large avocados, halved and pitted
- Salt and black pepper to taste
- 2 teaspoons lemon juice

Marinade:

- 2 lbs. shrimp, peeled and deveined
- 2 garlic cloves, minced
- 1 1/2 teaspoon salt
- 1/2 teaspoon cayenne pepper
- 1 teaspoon paprika
- 3 tablespoons olive oil
- 1 tablespoon lemon juice

Preparation:

1. Mix shrimp with garlic, salt, cayenne pepper, paprika, olive oil and lemon juice.
2. Cover and leave this marinade for 30 minutes.

3. Mash avocado with black pepper and salt in a bowl.

4. At medium-high heat, preheat your grill.

5. Grill the shrimp in the grill for 3 minutes per side.

6. Set the cucumber slices on the serving platter.

7. Top these slices with avocado mash and place a grilled shrimp on top.

8. Enjoy.

Serving Suggestion: Serve the bites with spinach or cream cheese dip.

Variation Tip: Add shredded parmesan on top.

Nutritional Information Per Serving:

Calories 82 | Fat 4g |Sodium 232mg | Carbs 7g | Fiber 1g | Sugar 0g | Protein 4g

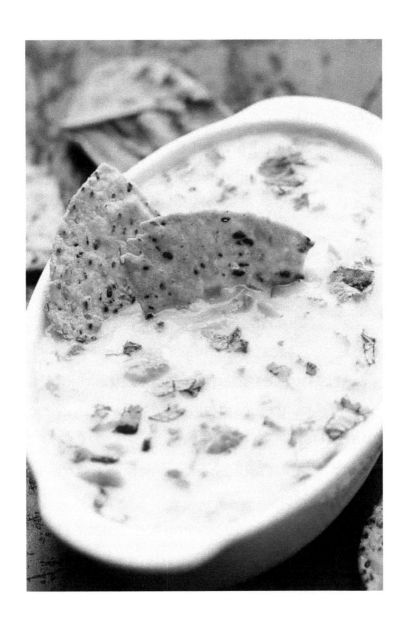

Queso Dip

Prep Time: 15 minutes.

Cook Time: 12 minutes.

Serves: 8

Ingredients:

- 1 lb. lean ground turkey
- 1 small onion diced
- 1 package. taco seasoning
- 2 tablespoons butter
- 2 ½ tablespoons flour
- 1 ½ cup milk
- 1/2 teaspoon salt
- 1/8 teaspoons black pepper
- 4 ounces sharp cheddar shredded
- 4 ounces can jalapeños drained, diced

Preparation:

1. Sauté turkey with onion in a large skillet until golden.
2. Add taco seasoning then mix well.
3. Sauté flour with butter in another pan for 2 minutes.
4. Remove it from the heat, pour in the milk and mix well until lump-free.

5.   Add cheddar cheese, black pepper and salt then mix well until melted.

6.   Stir in turkey meat mixture and diced jalapenos.

7.   Serve warm.

Serving Suggestion: Serve the dip with zucchini fries.

Variation Tip: Add olive slices or tomato salad on top.

Nutritional Information Per Serving:

Calories 229 | Fat 5g |Sodium 510mg | Carbs 37g |
Fiber 5g | Sugar 4g | Protein 11g

Peanut Butter Cookies

Prep Time: 15 minutes.

Cook Time: 12 minutes.

Serves: 4

Ingredients:

- 4 sachets Lean & Green silky peanut butter shake
- 1/4 teaspoon baking powder
- 1/4 cup unsweetened almond milk
- 1 tablespoon butter, melted
- 1/4 teaspoon vanilla extract
- 1/8 teaspoon salt

Preparation:

1. At 350 degrees F, preheat your oven.
2. Mix baking powder with peanut butter fueling in a bowl.
3. Stir in vanilla extract, melted butter, and almond milk, then mix until smooth.
4. Divide the dough into 8 cookies and place in a baking sheet, lined with parchment paper.
5. Flatten the cookies and bake for 12 minutes in the preheated oven.
6. Allow the cookies to cool and serve.

Serving Suggestion: Serve the cookies with pure maple or apple sauce.

Variation Tip: Drizzle maple syrup on top before serving.

Nutritional Information Per Serving:

Calories 201 | Fat 7g |Sodium 269mg | Carbs 35g | Fiber 4g | Sugar 12g | Protein 6g

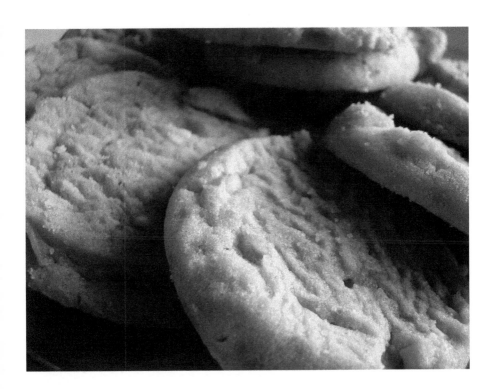

Goat Cheese Crostini

Prep Time: 15 minutes.

Cook Time: 10 minutes.

Serves: 2

Ingredients:

- 1 baguette
- 4-ounce goat cheese
- Honey
- Fresh mint, chopped
- Ground black pepper

Preparation:

1. At 350 degrees F, preheat your oven.
2. Cut the baguette into thin slices, diagonally.
3. Place the baguette slices in a baking sheet and bake for 10 minutes.
4. Divide goat cheese, honey, herbs, and black pepper on top of the bread slices.
5. Enjoy.

Serving Suggestion: Serve the crostini with chilli garlic sauce.

Variation Tip: Add sliced olives to the topping.

Nutritional Information Per Serving:

Calories 348 | Fat 12g |Sodium 710mg | Carbs 44g | Fiber 5g | Sugar 3g | Protein 11g

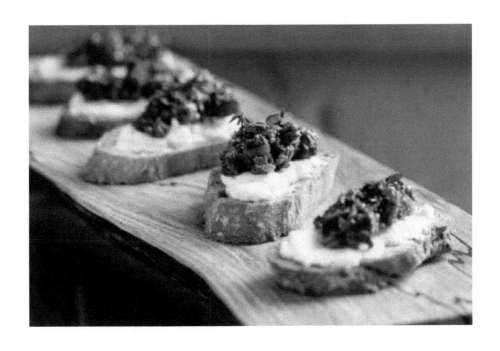

Buffalo Cauliflower

Prep Time: 15 minutes.

Cook Time: 36 minutes.

Serves: 4

Ingredients:

Buffalo cauliflower

- 1 head cauliflower
- 2 tablespoons olive oil
- ½ teaspoon kosher salt

Buffalo sauce

- 2 tablespoons unsalted butter
- 1 garlic clove
- ¼ cup Frank's hot sauce

Blue cheese sauce

- 1 cup plain yogurt
- ½ cup blue cheese crumbles
- 1/4 teaspoon salt
- 1 teaspoon garlic powder
- Fresh ground black pepper
- Celery, to serve

Preparation:

1. At 450 degrees F, preheat your oven.

2. Cut the cauliflower head into small florets and toss them with salt and olive oil on a baking sheet.

3. Bake the cauliflower for 35 minutes in the preheated oven.

4. For buffalo sauce, sauté garlic with butter in a saucepan for 30 seconds.

5. Stir in hot sauce and sauté for 30 seconds.

6. Toss in the cauliflower florets and mix well with the sauce.

7. For cheese dip, blend all its ingredients in a blender.

8. Serve the cauliflower with cream cheese dip.

9. Enjoy.

Serving Suggestion: Serve the florets with tomato ketchup.

Variation Tip: Coat the cauliflower in breadcrumbs before cooking.

Nutritional Information Per Serving:

Calories 175 | Fat 16g |Sodium 255mg | Carbs 31g | Fiber 1.2g | Sugar 5g | Protein 4.1g

Peanut Butter Brownie

Prep Time: 15 minutes.

Cook Time: 1 minute.

Serves: 4

Ingredients:

- 3 tablespoons peanut butter powder
- 3 tablespoons water
- 6 packets Lean & Green double chocolate brownie fueling
- 1 cup of water

Preparation:

1. Mix peanut butter powder with water and chocolate brownie in a bowl.
2. Divide this batter on a baking sheet lined with parchment paper into small mounds.
3. Cover and freeze for 40 minutes.
4. Serve.

Serving Suggestion: Serve the brownies with chocolate dip.

Variation Tip: Dip the brownies in white chocolate syrup.

Nutritional Information Per Serving:

Calories 361 | Fat 10g |Sodium 218mg | Carbs 56g | Fiber 10g | Sugar 30g | Protein 14g

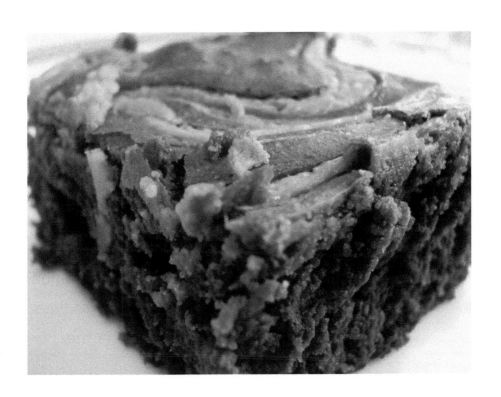

Chocolate Cherry Cookie

Prep Time: 15 minutes.

Cook Time: 12 minutes.

Serves: 4

Ingredients:

- 1 Lean & Green dark chocolate covered cherry shake
- ½ teaspoons baking powder
- 2 tablespoons water

Preparation:

1. At 350 degrees F, preheat your oven.
2. Mix cherry shake with water and baking powder in a bowl.
3. Divide this batter on a baking sheet, lined with parchment paper, into 8 small cookies.
4. Bake these cookies 12 minutes in the preheated oven.
5. Serve.

Serving Suggestion: Serve the cookies with fresh berries on top.

Variation Tip: Add cherry preserves at the centre of the cookies.

Nutritional Information Per Serving:

Calories 118 | Fat 20g |Sodium 192mg | Carbs 23.7g | Fiber 0.9g | Sugar 19g | Protein 5.2g

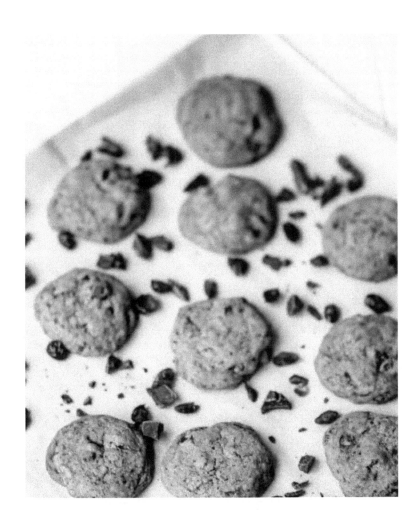

Stuffed pears with almonds

Prep Time: 15 minutes.

Cook Time: 25 minutes.

Serves: 6

Ingredients:

Spices

- 4 pinches cinnamon
- 3 ounces flour
- 3 ounces granulated sugar
- 2 tablespoons soup brown sugar
- 3 ounces almonds, powdered
- 1 ½ ounces frilled almond
- 1 ½ ounces hazelnut
- 3 ½ ounces butter
- 6 pears

Preparation:

1. Mix butter with cinnamon, sugars, flour, almonds, hazelnut in a food processor.
2. Core the pears and divide the nuts mixture into these pears.
3. Place the stuffed pears on a baking sheet.
4. Bake these pears for 25 minutes in the oven at 300 degrees F.
5. Serve once cooled.

Serving Suggestion: Serve the pears with a scoop of vanilla cream on top.

Variation Tip: Add chopped pecans to the filling as well.

Nutritional Information Per Serving:

Calories 248 | Fat 16g |Sodium 95mg | Carbs 38.4g | Fiber 0.3g | Sugar 10g | Protein 14.1g

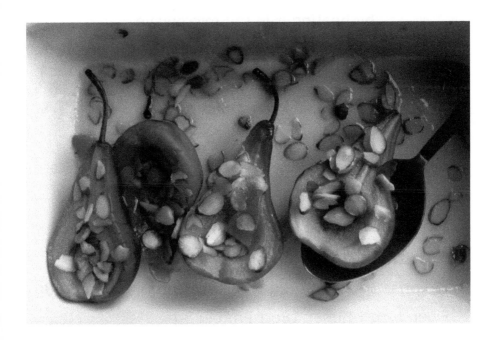

Peanut Butter Cups

Prep Time: 15 minutes.

Cook Time: 12 minutes.

Serves: 4

Ingredients:

- 1/4 cup creamy peanut butter
- 5 ounces chocolate
- Cacao Nibs, Sea Salt

Preparation:

1. Melt chocolate with peanut butter in a bowl by heating it in the microwave.
2. Mix well and divide this mixture into 12 mini muffin cups.
3. Cover and refrigerate for 1 hour.
4. Serve.

Serving Suggestion: Serve the cups with chocolate or apple sauce.

Variation Tip: Dip the bites in white chocolate syrup.

Nutritional Information Per Serving:

Calories 117 | Fat 12g |Sodium 79mg | Carbs 24.8g | Fiber 1.1g | Sugar 18g | Protein 5g

Medifast Rolls

Prep Time: 15 minutes.

Cook Time: 35 minutes.

Serves: 4

Ingredients:

- 3 eggs, separated
- 3 tablespoons cream cheese
- Pinch cream of tartar
- 1 packet Splenda

Preparation:

1. At 350 degrees F, preheat your oven.
2. Beat separated egg whites with cream of tartar in a bowl until fluffy.
3. Blend yolks with Splenda and cream cheese in a bowl until pale.
4. Fold in egg whites and mix gently.
5. Layer a baking sheet with parchment paper.
6. Divide the batter onto the baking sheet into cookie rounds.
7. Bake these rolls for 35 minutes in the oven at 350 degrees F.
8. Serve once cooled.

Serving Suggestion: Serve the rolls with creamy frosting on top.

Variation Tip: Add chopped pecans or walnuts to the batter.

Nutritional Information Per Serving:

Calories 195 | Fat 3g |Sodium 355mg | Carbs 20g | Fiber 1g | Sugar 25g | Protein 1g

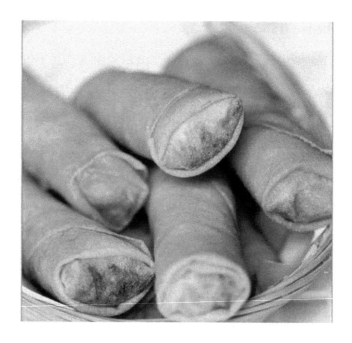